Eat and get Thin with Intermittent Fasting

Discover how to Burn Fat, Lose Weight and Get in the Best Shape of Your Life with Intermittent Fasting and the Detox Diet

The following Book is reproduced below with the goal of providing information that is as accurate and reliable as possible. Regardless, purchasing this Book can be seen as consent to the fact that both the publisher and the author of this book are in no way experts on the topics discussed within and that any recommendations or suggestions that are made herein are for entertainment purposes only. Professionals should be consulted as needed prior to undertaking any of the action endorsed herein.

This declaration is deemed fair and valid by both the American Bar Association and the Committee of Publishers Association and is legally binding throughout the United States.

Furthermore, the transmission, duplication, or reproduction of any of the following work including specific information will be considered an illegal act irrespective of if it is done electronically or in print. This extends to creating a secondary or tertiary copy of the work or a recorded copy and is only allowed with an expressed written consent from the Publisher. All additional right reserved.

The information in the following pages is broadly considered to be a truthful and accurate account of facts, and as such any inattention, use, or misuse of the information in question by the reader will render any resulting actions solely under their purview. There are no scenarios in which the publisher or the original author of this work can be in any fashion deemed liable for any hardship or damages that may befall them after undertaking information described herein.

Additionally, the information in the following pages is intended only for informational purposes and should thus be thought of as universal. As befitting its nature, it is presented without assurance regarding its prolonged validity or interim quality. Trademarks that are mentioned are done without written consent and can in no way be considered an endorsement from the trademark holder.

Table of Contents

Introduction

Congratulations on purchasing this book and thank you for doing so. The world of diet is growing increasingly chaotic, and downloading this book is the first step you can take towards actually doing something about healthful dieting. The first step is also not always the easiest, which is why the information you find in the following chapters is so important to take to heart as they are not concepts that can be put into action immediately. If you file these concepts away for when you need them, when the time comes to actually use them, you will be glad you have them at hand.

To that end, the following chapters will discuss the primary preparedness principals that you will need to consider if you ever hope to realistically be ready for losing weight and gain health with a healthy intermittent fasting diet. This means you will want to consider the quality of your food including the potential issues raised by their quality, how they can best be utilized in a meal and various tools you might need to keep your mind focused on the task at hand.

With quality out of the way, you will then learn everything you need to know about preparing a wide variety of recipes including common fruit and vegetable recipes along with less common dishes as well. Rounding out the three primary requirements for successful dieting, you will then learn about crucial food storage principles and what they will mean for you. Finally, you will learn how building a diet plan is likely the best choice for realizing all your hard work.

I am happy to welcome you to the world of the intermittent fasting and to help you lose weight, change your life, and become a healthier person.

Chapter 1: A recurring problem

In this day and age, the phenomenon of obesity is an increasing trend not only among adults but in children as well; This is why, interest and sensitivity towards this problem have increased both from a strictly medical point of view and from a social point of view as well. This is the reason why a lot of experts call this new health awareness movement, the "healthy eating" culture.

Eating and drinking are the response to physiological and physical drives through which the body requires energy and nourishment. Eating and drinking, however, also represent a psychological experience, which corresponds to the fulfillment of a desire. So the food takes on values that go well beyond the simple nourishment of the body. In fact, there has always been a broader conception of food, linked to social, cultural and symbolic factors that derive in turn from the habits and customs, from history, and from the values that characterize a given society. If it is true that nutrition is a physiological necessity, it is also true that the answers to the latter are conditioned by the socio-cultural context and can be considered social and cultural responses.

This explains why in many cases obesity does not depend on organic factors but is linked to an alteration of dietary behavior of psychological origin.

Psychological support therefore becomes a very important element in the management and treatment of the obese patient, since the psychicological factors can affect both the causes and the effects and have relevant consequences for the body.

With respect to the psychological causes, food can become a substance that creates psychological dependency. In fact, it is not uncommon to see it working as a refuge or as an analgesic substance against the sufferings experienced on a daily basis, or against complex situations. Therefore moods like anxiety, depression, stress, emotional inhibition can affect the relationship with food and cause weight gain.

Often the food is not tasted, but gobbled up to quickly fill an oppressive sense of inner emptiness, confused with the feeling of real hunger. Eating, or rather binge eating, then, can become, the only indiscriminate response to emotional and psychological issues. Food can compensate for a lack of care and self love, it can temporarily attenuate anxiety states or depressive symptoms, it can console us with disappointments, failures or even traumatic events (such as grief, separations and many other psychological issues). Anger, tension, boredom and other emotions are often confused with hunger.

The origins of what is described can be traced in the type of relationship established between the child and his first maternal and paternal figures, a relationship that is also mediated by the ways in which the food aspect is treated during the early stages of life. A common feature of mothers with young babies that suffer from obesity is precisely that of having imposed their concept of nutrition on their children compared to what would have been their actual needs. If the mother nourishes the child on the basis of their own convictions and beliefs, such as the one according to which a fat child is a beautiful and healthy child, or the one according to which food must be supplied according to precise patterns in terms of quantity, quality and schedules, this mother does not take into account the actual and physiological needs of the child. Over time the child, having difficulty in perceiving the internal state of need and desire, will begin to nourish himself depending mainly on external signals and factors.

It may also happen that the mother is emotionally distant from the child while being very present with respect to her task or role. The child can then perceive food as a method to escape self love problems and, as an adult, can keep eating in the same way. This causes emotions to be channeled only through food and the psychic processing of discomfort is replaced by the gratification that comes from external sensations. Also the presence of a strong symbiotic bond with the mother during childhood can be a predisposing factor to obesity. The child's dependence constraint on the mother, which in the beginning is of course functional to the child's survival, if it is not replaced by a progressive separation and individuation processes, which allow the individual's psychological growth in terms of autonomy, can cause a lot of damage going on. In fact, if this does not happen, it does not leave enough space for the child to become psychologically mature and an independent individual, able to make his own choices. Often the child is considered a precious asset to which the best care is needed but at the same time his individuality is not recognized.

11

Not only that, but in this way the child is not able to face and tolerate common problems; therefore in the future it will be difficult to delay the satisfaction of a need, which is instead a typical ability of A psychologically mature individual.

Even if we decide to avoid generalizations, however, it should be underlined that the dynamics that come into play when it comes to obesity are highly subjective, and even the reference to early childhood experiences acquires a certain relevance and meaning only if we refer to models of relationship between the child and his maternal and paternal figures. This is to say that there is not a "one size fits all" reason for obesity, but that a lot of the times it can be predicated to the parents' teachings about nutrition.

Feelings of guilt, depressive symptoms and low self-esteem are the main psychological issues found in the obese person.

Depressive symptoms can result from the inability to observe a strict diet combined with experiencing numerous failures. Depressive experiences can be so significant that they ca interfere with the quality of life of the individual as a whole. Unfortunately a lot of patients tend to use food as an escape and this makes everything worse.

How does low self-esteem cause nutritional disorders? Low self-esteem is found to the in those individuals that tend to overestimate the appearance of their body, placing in the achievement of a better physical form unrealistic expectations of personal affirmation and social consensus. Not only that though. In fact, during the evolution of the disease, the obese can progressively lose his self-esteem because of possible failures in weight loss attempts This is something that a lot of doctors tend to avoid when they are working with a patients, because of the psychological harm that can be done if the first attempts at losing the extra weight do not go as planned.. In fact, a failure can cause a vicious circle which makes the patient eat more when he fails at losing weight.

Besides trying to solve medical problems caused by the extra weight, what motivates the patient to decide for a treatment of obesity is a generalized discomfort. In fact, a lot of patients say they feel "not normal", "different" or even "socially discriminated" because of their weight, which creates significant obstacles both psychological and physical. This leads them to perceive their body as "stranger", or "without borders" and reject it with consequent difficulties in social relationships and self-acceptance.

In the treatment of obesity, the primary goal is not to lose weight but to acquire a renewed and healthy lifestyle and eating habits. After this has been accomplished there is the opportunity for of an approach marked not only by the medical / dietary aspect but also by the attention to the psycho-educational as well. In other words, before addressing the psychological issue, it is important to work on learning the right eating habits. At the beginning of the therapy, for example, sensitization groups are very useful, since they allow the patient to achieve a progressive awareness of their psychological distress and give motivation to those patients who, coming from numerous failed attempts at treatment, define themselves as lacking possibility of change. In these groups, through the comparison with others who share similar symptoms and experiences, in a caring environment, it is easier for the patient to verbalize their painful experiences and to put his feelings into words. By becoming aware of how much the symptom can also limit someone's life, the patient rediscovers his needs and desires that can thus become a drive for a positve change.

In conclusion, the therapeutic process, that takes all these factors into account, should not only have the aim of restoring organic integrity to the individual as it was before the pathology. Instead, it should tend towards a more complete evolution of the person, in the direction of a constant process of change and oriented to the acquisition of a new awareness of oneself and of one's own unconscious mechanisms of relationship with food. Only by creating positive habits it is possible to become healthier.

Food is a fundamental element of the life of each individual and is heavily loaded with meanings: dining in company build our relationships, the choice of food expresses who we are and has the power to change our mood in a matter of seconds. But food also has a dark side: when we eat excessively we are preoccupied with being fat. Thus, eating can easily turn from a moment of delightful pleasure to one of indigestion.

In recent years, there have been a lot of interesting researches about the power of food on the human mind. Here are the most interesting studies.

1. DOES SIZE MATTER?

We usually think that the amount of food we eat depends on how hungry we are. It is certainly a factor, but it is not the only one. We are also influenced, for example, by the size of the plate and its presentation, as demonstrated in a study by Wansink and collaborators (2005). The participants were simply asked to eat a soup. In the middle of action the plate was "magically" filled a little at a time by a small tube placed under the table, without people noticing. Others were served a portion of soup in the classic way. Both groups, therefore, ate the same ration of soup, but one group was convinced that it had eaten a smaller portion. This group reported being more hungry and less satiated than the other. The researchers explained that this result may be due to the fact that our stomach gives raw information about how much we eat, while it is the sight to tell us if we have eaten so much or little and to help determine our feeling of satiety.

2. NEVER EAT ALONE

Eating together has surprising positvie psychological effect. In fact, as humans, we tend to give eating a strong social connotation Recent studies have shown that by eating with other people that do not suffer from eating disorders, people who suffered from obesity tended to choose healthier food than when nobody was around. This is why eating with someone you admire or in a healthy context can be beneficial when dealing with eating disorders.

3. THE TASTE GETS WORSE WITH AGE

With age, taste becomes gradually weaker. One study noted that, above all, the ability to perceive salt deteriorated considerably over the years (Mojet et al., 2001). Depending on the type of taste (sweet, salty, sour, bitter) elderly people need to season between 2 and 9 times more to perceive the same taste when they were young. Men seem to be more affected by the loss of this sense.

4. GREAT WAITER = GREAT CUSTOMER

In a recent research, McFerran and his collaborators (2010) observed how the choice of the dish at the restaurant varies depending on whether it is served by a fat or a thin waiter. Healthy people choose more caloric dishes if they are recommended by fat waiters, as they feel unconsciously authorized because they see people fatter than them. Non-healthy people, on the other hand, choose more caloric dishes if they are recommended by lean waiters, as lean people tend to be more persuasive.

5. YOU BECOME THE UNION OF YOUR 5 CLOSEST FRIENDS

It is very likely that having fat friends will lead us to gain weight. Christakis and his collaborators (2007) found that the probability of gaining weight for people with obese friends increases by 57%. This is due to the fact that people are strongly influenced by the behaviors they repeatedly observe. People eat a lot more if those who eat eat a lot, while they eat less if they are surrounded by friends who eat little. Women seem to be more susceptible to this behavior. Furthermore, the influence of society also plays an important role: it is customary to think that men must eat much more than women.

6. EAT WITH ATTENTION

Eating can become an automatic routine: when you have lunch or dinner, your mind usually wanders. When people are distracted, such as by TV or because they are talking, they eat a lot more (Bolhuis et al., 2013). When we are not focused on food, we tend to eat more but also to experience less pleasure in doing so. That's why a useful strategy in weight control protocols is to pay close attention to everything you eat and the way you eat. For example, small and slow bites are recommended. In this way, not only do people eat less, they find more pleasure in eating as well.

7. DO YOU WANT A SMOKED SALMON ICE CREAM?

Food labels create specific expectations, which in turn influence the taste of food. For example, putting funny names on the bottles has the magic power to make the wine contained in them better. In another study on the subject, Yeomans and his collaborators (2008) had a smoked salmon mousse tasted in a sample of subjects. Half of the participants were told it was a mousse, at the other half were told it was ice cream. The subjects who thought they were eating ice-cream reported how awful the tasted food was, unlike the others, who instead considered the delicious mousse. So: putting funny labels on food can increase its attractiveness, however, attentive to the expectations that these labels arouse, as they may be disappointed.

8. THE DANGER OF EMOTIONAL HUNGER

With "emotional hunger" we refer to the idea that all emotions, and not just rabies, can influence eating behavior. It is usually observed that people tend to look for more sugary and fatty foods when they are in a bad mood. Furthermore, negative emotions encourage one to prefer continuous snacks rather than a complete meal, and to avoid vegetables. Unfortunately, good mood does not necessarily make us eat healthy foods.

9. WE TEND TO EAT WHAT OTHER PEOPLE ORDER AT A RESTAURANT

Have you ever had dinner in a restaurant with a group of people, to choose a dish and then to change your mind by hearing other people order the same thing you wanted to order? According to a study by Ariely & Levav (2000), it happens much more often than we think. The cause of this behavior is that we want to bring out our individuality. The funny thing, however, is that the authors have found that people like their second choice less than the first. Sometimes, wanting to stand out only to feel unique can be backfired. So: order only the dishes that you really like!

10. I AM EATING AN IDEA AND IT IS TASTY

What strange foods did you eat? Fried bats or tarantulas, grasshoppers or tuna eyes?

Surely you have already been involved in this kind of conversation. People begin to list all sorts of exotic foods they've tried competing for those who have tasted the weirdest dish. We do not eat only food, but ideas as well. People know, for example, that bacon ice cream will have a particular flavor, but by trying it they gain an unusual experience. It's not just a reason to brag, people love the idea of trying new experiences. It is a question of enriching one's self-image. People want to see each other, and be seen, as interesting subjects who choose varied and extravagant experiences.

Chapter 2: How to develop a healthy relationship with food

Each person has a different relationship with food and with the act of eating. Sometimes the boundary between a healthy relationship with food and a problematic one can be very little and overcoming it can be a matter of a small effort. To establish a healthy relationship with food, it may be useful to take as an example those who already have a powerful relationship with food. If you do not know anybody that is really into eating healthy, we recommend you to follow these tips.

- They eat consciously: the body has its own intrinsic wisdom, knows when to eat, how much and when to stop. People who have a healthy relationship with food rely on their senses rather than what they think or others say. According to Magrette Fletcher of the Center for Mindful Eating eating consciously (mindful eating) can help to recognize the body's responses to food without judging it with the mind

- They allow themselves a little of everything, albeit in

moderation: according to Edward Abramson, author of "Emotional Eating", foods are not intrinsically good or bad, but the experience we have with them is not. It is our categorical judgment that creates real hardship. Recognizing which foods and consumption situations we like gives us valuable insights into our future choices. People with a healthy relationship with food think that eating is an opportunity for themselves to nourish and take care of their body, they do not live that moment as a duty to lean towards a food or another

- They know the right time to eat: people who have a balanced relationship with food are aware of the hunger they have, why they are attracted to one food or another, which is why they hardly exceed. Such people know from experiences that if they come from a long period of deprivation of a food that they like very much, it is easier for them to exceed

- They eat when they are physically hungry: eating motivated by emotional motivations, usually triggered by anxiety, stress, depression, anger, can induce to binge, especially foods rich in fats, sugars and calories in quantities much greater than the real needs of the body. People balanced in their relationship with food eat when their body requires food

- They stop eating when they are pleasantly sated: hunger and sense of satiety arise gradually and are gradually accentuated. There are people who are not aware of these stimuli until they become very accentuated. Mindfulness or awareness helps us to be aware of even the most subtle clues so we can satisfy them before they become too accentuated and expose us to the risk of binging ourselves

- They eat breakfast: according to Marjorie Nolan Cohn of the Academy of Nutrition & Dietetics, people who regularly eat breakfast in a healthy and complete way seem to have more energy, attention, memory, lower levels of cholesterol than those who do not consume it. In addition they are thinner and overall have better health than those who do not eat breakfast. A balanced breakfast provides a balance between carbohydrates, proteins, fats, without exceeding with simple sugars to avoid glycemic peaks

- They do not keep junk food at home: the moment

you are aware of your own patterns, habits, food preferences and above all emotional reactions related to food, you can change them in a practical way. A useful strategy may be the one that does not keep the so-called junk food at home that usually generates greater temptations, feelings of guilt, and subsequent relapses, both for the mental and emotional experiences that triggers, and for the biochemical reactions to which gives rise

- Do not sit with a whole package of food: if, for example, we like a certain type of ice cream, it may be useful to serve a portion in a cup and carefully place the rest in the freezer, or use sealed portions. If, on the other hand, you keep in front of the multi-portion packs you risk triggering the one-bite mechanism pulls the other. Some foods, in particular, are particularly likely to elicit such a reaction

- They know the difference between a snack and a whim: a snack is a small break between one meal and another. It's a way to fill your stomach a little so as not to get too hungry for the next meal. The choice of snack is crucial to continue in your healthy and balanced diet. A whim, however, is a pure fun, pleasure, mostly independent of hunger. It is not to be condemned in absolute terms, the important thing is awareness.

- They are allowed to enjoy food: often food and the act of eating take place on their feet, in front of a computer, in a car, in a hurry, without paying particular attention. People who have a healthy and balanced relationship with food take in the right time, calm, attention, space to eat. Nursing, in fact, is not only a merely physical act, but also mental and emotional, and these people are aware of it

- They do not compensate for meals: when you feel guilty about something you have eaten, there is often an instinct to compensate for your intake by doing extra exercises at the gym, or skipping the next meal. On the contrary, the more balanced people, when they decide to eat something more or more substantial at a meal, in the following or the previous one are kept lighter, but they do not restrict their diet to the point of falling victim to a binge in following. The balance of food intake seems to be healthy if distributed over a week, you can not expect to limit it to a day

- They do not eat to see the scaling needle going down: people with a good relationship with food eat for the pleasure of eating, of feeling good, not for other purposes. When the focus shifts to other ends, especially weight loss, it risks to subtract part of the intrinsic pleasure linked to food and introduces a thought that risks becoming an obsession

- They are not afraid of feeling hungry: people who do not have a good relationship with food are often afraid of feeling hungry because they feel the real risk of overeating and above all of getting fat. People aware of their body, their instincts, and what foods are good for their body, are well tolerated, they know how to adjust accordingly

- Their interest in food does not interfere with their daily lives: there are people for whom their attention to food, both the junk and the healthy, is such as to monopolize all their thoughts and activities of the day. Being too rigid and normative in your approach to food can cause personal and relational problems just like having no rules does. To understand if our relationship with food is well integrated with our life or not, it can be useful to observe if it interferes with daily activities, work, friendships, affections or if it is compatible with them.

Chapter 3: Overcoming emotional eating issues

Common sense tells us that to be fit we have to eat less and exercise more, but this is easier said than done. Everyone knows the golden rules for a healthy and active lifestyle, but despite this awareness sometimes one feels stuck, unable to carry out the good intentions.

Generally good initial intentions give way to a sense of discouragement in the face of the difficulty in carrying forward the set goals. In this way, instead of feeling better, we become more and more pessimistic, sad and disappointed by ourselves.

We spend hours worrying about the future by pitying ourselves for what we have or have not eaten and how long we have been inactive in the past. A battle that exhausts us and that has the sole purpose of making us completely lose the present moment, the only one in which we really have the power to change the course of our lives.

Only we can decide to put an end to this struggle and to do so we must learn not to lose ourselves again in regrets.

Every minute spent worrying about what could have been or evaluating what may happen is a minute that we lose in our rendezvous with life, a lost opportunity to engage in activities that we like and make us feel good.

Being fully and consciously present in every single moment is called Mindfulness, an approach to life that helps us to live the present and that, when applied to the field of nutrition, provides us with useful tools to control how much and what we eat.

Being Mindful means being totally conscious and aware of what is in and around us, in every single moment, without judgment or prejudice, stopping our thoughts and concerns. By focusing on these statements it becomes possible to approach the food in a different way, becoming aware of every bite.

Mindful Eating

Mindful eating has these characteristics:

- Choose what you want to eat carefully, without letting the rush replace you;

- Be aware of the fact that you are going to eat, avoiding distractions that would make this condition difficult, like watching television, reading, working on a computer;

- Before starting to eat stop for a moment to become aware of where you are, of the food in front of you. You can do it by taking a couple of deep breaths. This allows you to reconnect to yourself for a conscious meal;

- Use all five senses. The food does not activate only the taste, but also the sight of touch, smell and hearing. Allowing you to enjoy what you are eating at 360 °;

- Serve your own serving of food in the dish directly from the beginning of the meal, so as to be aware of what is the amount of food you are about to eat. This also helps in containing portions that could become excessive by using them several times;

- Taste small quantities and chew the food for a long time, so as to fully enjoy what you eat;

- Eat slowly, calmly and relaxed. In this way there is awareness of the signals that the body sends to us, stopping at the first sense of satiety.

- The distractions and the frenzy in everyday life reinforce the habit of ingesting food without thinking and this increases the possibility of gaining weight or not feeling good about yourself.

Developing a good relationship with food is possible by learning to self-regulate and becoming aware of the thoughts and emotions that are related to our eating behavior.

With care and practice it is possible to become more aware of our eating and our lives, adequately nourishing both our body and our mind.

Chapter 4: The solution to eat and get thin: intermittent fasting

Intermittent fasting is one of the latest "fads" in terms of nutrition aimed at weight loss and muscle anabolism. A trend that seems to be able to impose itself in this and in the coming seasons, opposing the previous currents of thought that, of course, are still pursued by the majority of sector aficionados.

One of the basic principles of traditional diet suggests losing weight by exploiting the c.d. ADS, or the specific dynamic action of food, or - better yet - the energy expenditure that is attributable to the digestive processes. In even clearer terms, it is thought that - with the same calories being introduced - it is better to try to divide the meals as much as possible, since in this way it is also possible to burn more energy for their digestion and absorption. In this way, we try to reduce the time laps on an empty stomach, avoiding the sensation of hunger. According to some scholars, in this way it can also promote the containment of cortisol, the hormone of stress and hunger, while maintaining the thyroid function. So a traditional approach, which was often combined with the need to support muscle growth: the prevailing opinion was (and is, for many) that of continuously nourishing the body.

The intermittent fasting was then opposed to the above mentioned approach, a principle that is often enunciated in a rather confused and unclear way. Someone suggests for example to binge as much as possible and then fast for one or two days, while others - less radical - propose a system with 16 hours of fasting and 8 hours in which 2 or 3 meals can be consumed.

Beyond this, the basic principle of intermittent fasting is to create a fasting period with a duration that can affect the overall caloric balance and hormone metabolism. Some scholars suggest that under conditions of "food abstinence", we would see the increase in IGF-1, or somatomedin, and would also help the secretion of GH, or somatropin, the growth hormone or well-being, which promotes lipolysis necessary for weight loss.

As obvious, the above indications are simply broad

statements about a diet that is particularly in vogue right now. However, we advise you not to proceed independently with this diet, but agree with your doctor every step to find a better well-being and a better shape.

The intermittent fasting regime is also a rather complex one, which deserves a personalized study with a specialist. For example, you can remember how despite the diet exploits the window of fasting, meals that are taken in the remaining period can not be consumed in freedom (otherwise you run the risk of affecting the sacrifices made in the part of the fast!). Furthermore, you must always try to combine the appropriate physical activity with this diet.

Therefore, the intermittent fasting protocol will be characterized by 3 daily meals and 1 training session, with a fasting window equal to 16 hours. The first meal should be eaten as soon as you get up, focusing on a few grams of fat and a lot of proteins and carbohydrates with a low glycemic index; the second meal must be a full breakfast; the third meal must immediately follow the training, and must be a complete meal. The fasting window will therefore start from

15 until the following morning.

Chapter 5: How does intermittent fasting work?

What is Intermittent Fasting and how is it useful? Does it help you to lose weight? Is it a good solution to increase muscle mass? And for weight loss? What is and how to do a body recomposition? Can intermittent fasting help you to live longer? Wait a minute: if you want the answer to these questions, you need to know how Intermittent Fasting works. The reason is simple:

Intermittent Fasting is no use if you do not understand how it works.

What is and how does Intermittent Fasting work?

Intermittent Fasting – IF - is a diet style that alternates between fasting and non-fasting periods. Nothing special, someone could say: when we sleep we fast everyone, and then eat when we wake up. So do we all do intermittent fasting?

Not really, since Intermittent Fasting has taken a separate

path: the phases of fasting and non-fasting are well studied and balanced to provide specific metabolic effects (in particular on what is called the "cellular energy sensor network"). It makes sure to burn fat in fasting and build muscle in nutrition.

Starting from scientific arguments, there have been created many models of intermittent fasting, which can be more or less valid. But the point remains the same:

Intermittent Fasting is no use if you do not understand how it works.

The goodness of Intermittent Fasting has been letting us unhook from schemes such as "do many small meals help to lose weight and increase the metabolic rate?". Disengaging from these patterns to engage with other schemes such as "I must necessarily fast 16 hours" is counterproductive. It is because eating feeling "forced" is always counterproductive.

So, how to get the advantages of Intermittent Fasting without having to face the disadvantages of "feeling compelled to diet"? Simple: you have to understand what

"Fasting" means.

The dictionary tells us that fasting represents abstention from food. But for the body we have to make distinctions.

- Real fasting: to abstain from food; that is, do not eat anything.
- Simulated fasting: make sure that the metabolic signals activated within the organism are the same ones that would activate in the abstention from food (metabolic fasting).
- Super fasting: activate those metabolic signals "of fasting" more powerfully than would occur in abstention from food.

But is it possible to simulate or even create conditions in which the organism is "more fasting" than it would be if it were in total abstinence from food? Yes, it is possible. Think of a fat burner (a weight-loss supplement). What does it do? It increases the metabolic rate and increases the energy expenditure. Which means that it determines a negative energy balance. If fasting is taken fat burner the body will more powerfully activate the metabolic pathways of "fasting" compared to the situation in which the fat burner is not taken.

The water would seem to do something similar, especially when drunk in a certain way (from 450-500 mL, as we will see shortly). Warning: the data do not report an increase in energy expenditure, but a transient lowering of the respiratory coefficient, which could reflect on the way in which the body uses the energy substrates (based, that is, more on the oxidation of fats).

To have good effects from Intermittent Fasting, simply do it!

1-2 complete meals have to be consumed in periods of greater relaxation; this is because the IF should make sure that the organism does not degenerate at the level of activation of the Autonomous Nervous System (divided into SNS, the one that makes us activate, and SNP, the one that makes us relax).

During the 24 hours, we pass through an active phase, in

which we are programmed to move and do activities, and a relaxation phase, in which we are programmed to digest, absorb and rest. Eating (a lot) during the active phase generates numbness, lethargy, and sleep at times when we should be active. This phase can be exploited by maximizing the effects of physiological activation, fasting, to improve metabolism and to oxidize (burn) more fat.

On the contrary, we can exploit the phase planned for us to digest and absorb, to make complete meals, improving absorption and more directing those nutrients towards the muscle tissue (especially if training has been done).

On the other hand, this kind of timing would seem to protect against fattening even if you eat badly.

Consume small, fat-based snacks when you are in a hurry or looking for greater focus, concentration, work or training abilities is a good idea. Basing these meals on fats is important to maintain optimal metabolic flexibility or mitochondrial function to burn fat efficiently (5). And of course, water. But not in small sips: better to drink "to boluses" of 400-500 mL every time you are thirsty or every

2-3 hours. The respiratory coefficient will be lowered, optimizing fat oxidation and mitochondrial function ("Super fasting").

A king's breakfast, a ladies' lunch, a poor dinner?

No, for most of us it is better to do the opposite. We all tend to be active during the day and tend to relax in the evening. Reason why it would be good to have a quick breakfast (or skip it altogether, beneficial in terms of metabolism and health).

"Yes but when? How long? And if it's hungry? Do you take a punch in the stomach until it passes? "Calm down.

Ask yourself, when you are hungry, "am I also tired?". This is a good way to start recognizing "true" hunger from "emotional" hunger (homeostatic vs hedonic). It would be good to start doing it.

The unresolved question remains that of the "complete meal". But what is meant by a complete meal? It depends on the food strategy you are following. Low carb? High Carb? Zone diet? CrossFit or Marathon athlete? Vegan or

Paleo?

The generic structure of meals in Intermittent Fasting is as follows (the sequence is not random):

- For starters, raw vegetables (a salad, for example); it would be a good idea to do it with every meal (it is not necessary to overdo and fill).
- Following, a quality protein source, such as meat, fish, eggs, or vegan alternatives if you follow a plant-based diet; this dish should be dosed to satisfy completely, but not to flood.
- Add mixed cooked vegetables, seasoned with oil / coconut oil / quality butter / seeds.

If the plan includes carbohydrates, it is better to introduce the carbohydrate plate after the protein one; the carbohydrate intake varies depending on the type of activity, the body type and lifestyle, as a starting point the volume of a punch is valid for the most part.

A "fine meal": for some it can be fruit, for other yogurt, for others still a piece of aged cheese, or even dark chocolate or dried fruit.

Apart from a first period, in which the schemes can regulate and make understand how certain mechanisms work, in the long term it is appropriate to try to find your own way. For example, if the moment of maximum relaxation is lunch, do not force yourself not to eat at that time to move all the nutrients to dinner. If, however, there are other reasons for keeping the most abundant dinner (How to stay with the family), the "simulated fasting" or the Temporary Glucidic Diet (see how in this guide) comes to help us.

By building the nutritional plan so that it includes a certain flexibility, it will be easier to stick to it over time on the basis of subjectivity and individual responses.

Chapter 6: The straight road to the body you deserve

When we want to lose a few extra pounds, we have a choice of diets to follow so vast that we often forget to understand how a diet really works and what are the risks and benefits it brings. One of the latest trends in the world of nutrition is intermittent fasting, very popular among athletes and considered by many to be one of the most effective methods to lose weight. We decided to explore the topic and share with you what we have discovered.

As suggested by the name itself, intermittent fasting is a model that alternates between periods of eating at periods when it is fasted. So this is not a real diet, but a food program that rather than suggesting what, tells you when to eat.

There are several methods of intermittent fasting and the most popular are:

- Scheme 16/8: also known as the leangains method.

This scheme divides the day into two parts: 8 hours in which you eat and 16 hours of fasting. It can be considered as an extension of the fast that is done automatically when you sleep, skipping breakfast and eating the first meal at noon and then eating until 8.00 in the evening.

- Every other day (5: 2): the idea of this model is that for two days a week the caloric intake is reduced to a maximum of 500/600 calories. The days do not have to be consecutive and on the other days you can eat whatever you want.

- Eat Stop Eat: according to this model you eat every other day, once or twice a week.

In every type of model you can drink low-calorie drinks.

Intermittent fasting goes beyond simple caloric restriction. Hormone balance is also changing, so that the body learns to make good use of fat reserves. Here are some important changes:

- Improves   insulin   sensitivity,   especially   in

combination with exercise. This point is very important for people who are trying to lose weight because if you have low insulin levels it is easier to burn fat. Studies have shown that overweight can affect insulin's ability to reduce blood sugar levels and as a result more insulin is released, further promoting fat storage.

- The secretion of growth hormone (GH) increases, accelerating protein synthesis so as to make fats available as an energy resource. Which means that you burn fat and get on muscles faster. In the bodybuilding world this hormone is taken in large quantities as a doping agent.

- Moreover, according to some studies, fasting activates autophagy, which removes damaged cells, contributes to cell renewal and generally supports regenerative processes.

By skipping meals, you create a caloric deficit and then you lose weight. Obviously, as long as you do not compensate for periods of fasting with foods high in sugar or fat, since this type of diet does not say exactly what you can and what you can not eat. Studies have shown that intermittent fasting, if done correctly, helps to prevent type 2 diabetes as well. In addition, the body learns to process the consumed food more efficiently. Some studies have also shown that a combination of strength training and the 16/8 method allows you to reduce a percentage of body fat greater than that which is eliminated only with training. So it seems to be very effective if combined with regular workouts.

Note: This type of diet is not particularly suitable for people suffering from diabetes or high blood pressure and for pregnant or nursing women. Before practicing this type of diet, it is better to consult a doctor.

Fasting can help you lose weight but if you are a person with an active social life, you have to take this into account when you decide to start this diet. Imagine some friends invite you to a Sunday birthday brunch. A delicious buffet with muesli, scrambled eggs, vegetables, salmon, all your friends are eating and you? There you are, drinking water because it is 10 and you can eat your first meal only at 12 o'clock. Plus dinner is scheduled for 7 in the evening. If programmed in advance, the diet allows you to eat with friends and relatives, but in general does not leave much room for flexibility and spontaneity.

Many people who follow this type of diet, complain of hunger attacks and a sense of fatigue, which can occur easily when you miss meals. Some say that once the critical phase has passed (about 2 days), the hunger disappears. At times when you feel a sense of hunger too strong, you can drink green tea or black coffee to be able to resist until the next meal.

Intermittent fasting is not for everyone, but it is a good way to reduce body fat. We must keep the food regime under control and avoid hamburgers, pizzas and fries. The goal remains to try to eat in a healthy way and to follow a balanced diet.

Chapter 7: The benefits of Intermittent Fasting

Would you like to live 100 years? Who would not want it after all?

An excellent practice of health and longevity is intermittent fasting, a food regimen in which you regularly eat a few days and take a break from food in others or for several hours of the day.

One of the errors of modern Western lifestyle is eating too often, which makes your body lazy in the repairing and renewal process of the cells.

Intermittent fasting very effectively mimics the eating habits of our ancestors, who did not have access to supermarkets and food or food at all times.

Alternating periods of eating until you reach satiety to periods of fasting is good. Modern research shows that these cycles are very beneficial: they improve cardiovascular health and metabolic functions and reduce the risks of cancer.

Intermittent fast renews the blood and the immune system

A study published in Cell Stem Cell found that intermittent fasting strengthens the immune system, which gets rid of damaged white blood cells and replaces them with new ones, causing stem cells to move from a state of "drowsiness and stasis" to a state renewal.

Fasting is essential to give your body a shock, to reset your body.

Researchers at the University of Southern California have discovered that during a prolonged period of fasting the white blood cells decrease, but when you start eating again, the number increases.

Further investigating this phenomenon, the researchers found that the body was eliminating old and damaged immune cells by replacing them with new cells.

The fasting cycle promotes regeneration through a key gene that controls the PKA enzyme.

During fasting, PKA is reduced, which starts the regeneration process that starts stem cells.

Scientists believe these findings have implications for

healthy aging and are trying to understand if these benefits also affect different systems and organs, beyond the immune system

Intermittent fasting is good for your heart, your brain and your waistline

Fasting has a very long history, has been used in various spiritual practices for millennia.

Today even the modern scientists tell us that fasting can have a great number of benefits, including the following:

It normalizes insulin and sensitivity to leptin and enhances the effectiveness and energy of mitochondria

One of the main mechanisms that make intermittent fasting so beneficial to health is related to the impact on sensitivity to insulin and leptin.

Sugar is a precious source of energy for your body, but if it is consumed continuously and in excessive quantities it causes resistance to insulin / leptin.

Insulin resistance / leptin is one of the main causes of chronic diseases such as heart disease, type 2

diabetes and cancer.

Intermittent fasting helps ensure that your body does not use sugars as a primary source of energy, but fats. Several evidences confirm that when your body adapts to burning fat instead of sugars, the risks of illness decrease significantly.

Intermittent fasting also normalizes ghrelin levels, known as the "hunger hormone". Another advantage of intermittent fasting is that it helps reduce the excessive craving of sugars.

Promotes the production of growth hormone (HGH)

Research has shown that fasting can increase HGH levels by 1,300% in women and 2,000 in men. HGH plays a very important role in health, physical activity and slows down the aging process.

It is also a fat burning hormone, which explains why fasting leads to weight loss.

It lowers triglyceride levels and improves biomarkers of other diseases

Reduces oxidative stress; Fasting decreases the

accumulation of oxidative radicals in cells, thus reducing the oxidative damage of cellular proteins, lipids and nucleic acids, associated with aging and disease.

Intermittent fasting protects your brain

Fasting stimulates the production of a protein called brain-derived neurotrophic factor (BDNF), which stimulates the release of new brain cells and numerous other compounds that protect you from Parkison and Alzheimer's.

The research suggests that fasting every other day (reducing your meals on the fasting day to 600 calories) can boost BDNF from 50 to 400%, depending on the region of the brain.

Animal research shows that fasting has a beneficial impact on longevity for different triggering mechanisms, including improved insulin sensitivity.

Intermittent fasting is one of the most effective ways to get rid of excess fats.

When your body does not need sugar as its primary source of energy, you experience a sense of hunger less than when your zuchero stores are quickly emptied.

Intermittent fasting and loss of lean mass

A side effect of intermittent fasting could be loss of lean mass.

However, Dr. Krista Varaday, assistant professor at Kinesiology and Nutrition at the University of Illinois, has conducted several studies on intermittent fasting and found that 90% of the weight that people lose is body fat, with only 10% of lean mass.

Being active and consuming the right amount of high quality protein helps reduce muscle mass loss.

Intermittent Fasting Plan 5: 2 by Dr. Michael Mosley

The term "intermittent fasting" covers a large number of food plans.

As a general rule, it involves cutting calories completely or in part, a couple of days a week, every day or even every day.

Dr. Michael Mosley is so convinced of the benefits of intermittent fasting that he wrote a book called *The Fast Diet: Lose Weight, Stay Healthy, and Live Longer with the Simple Secret of Intermittent Fasting.*

The fasting plan he proposed is to eat normally for 5 days a week and then to fast for two days, the intermittent fasting plan 5: 2.

During the days of fasting it is recommended to reduce the usual caloric intake to 1/4 or 600 calories for men and 500 calories for women, besides drinking water and tea.

It does not really matter which days you choose to fast. Monday is a good day to start, especially if you've had a very calories weekend.

On the day of fasting you can choose to distribute the 500/600 calories throughout the day or fast all day and make a single meal in the evening. Find the routine that's right for you.

Dr. Mosley gives 3 golden rules for a successful outcome:

1. Try to be sensitive on non-fasting days. Eat normally, give yourself good meals, but do not overdo it.

2. Pay attention to what you drink. Juices, milk, alcohol and smoothies usually contain many calories and sugars but do not satisfy your appetite.

3. Try adding another day of fasting. Try the 4: 3 plan (four days of normal eating and 3 days of calorie reduction). Or try fasting every other day, which will really kick your weight loss within a few months, especially if you exercise.

How to make the best fast. My 6 personal warnings

Fasting is not suitable for everyone because, by releasing many toxins, at first it can cause discomfort.

For some people it would be better to start to clean up some food before thinking about making a drastic fast, because this would lighten more and would not suddenly get to a fast that puts too many toxins in circulation, more than they would manage to to bear.

Intermittent fasting is not for everyone because it can sharpen the tendency to dehydration.

If you have swelling (which can also be just abdominal swelling), aching joints, exaggerated thinness, memory that is already beginning to run low, fasting could be counterproductive to your body.

It could give agitation, nervousness, a feeling of prostration, exaggerated fatigue, a swelling even greater than what you had.

To fast the intestine must be very efficient.
If you are constipated, it is best that you unblock the intestine completely before dedicating yourself to a fasting practice, in order to favor a correct elimination of waste and toxins.

Fasting must be gradual, especially if you've never done it.
You can approach the practice of fasting by starting to skip a meal and doing a little one-day fast to try and see how it goes.

A constant supply of liquids is needed on the day of fasting.
Do not do fasts without water, water is essential!
It takes liquids and it is necessary that these liquids are hot.
And then, depending on your constitution, you can

introduce centrifuged or take broths of very spicy vegetables.

Fasting should not be the excuse to binge on other days

Pay attention that the desire to make fast does not hide an inability to establish good constant habits. It does not have to be the punishment for getting rid of on other days.

Guidelines for fasting

1. Fast during a period of time when you can rest without stress
2. Always drink a lot during the fast, better if hot water
3. Continue doing the oil pulling and maybe take half a teaspoon of wheat grass in the morning
4. Be careful to always empty the intestine and, if necessary, help with the herbs. Mainly use raw centrifuged drinks (if you have heat symptoms) or hot soups with seaweed (if you have cold constitution)
5. You can introduce a couple of tablespoons a day of coconut oil, to nourish yourself without gaining weight.

6. You can do one day of fasting a week, but the most precious and powerful thing is to introduce a little daily fast. For some it is good in the morning and for others in the evening. Find out what the fast is for you.

7. Avoid the non-virtuous spiral of "intoxicating first and fasting later" because it is not healthy

8. Fasting mobilizes many toxins, so it could give you headaches and other symptoms of strong purification (halitosis, rashes on the skin, etc.)

There are some particular categories that should avoid fasting.

If you suffer from one of those conditions, focus on improving your nutrition before thinking about fasting:

1. Hypoglycemia;
2. Diabetes;
3. Chronic stress;
4. Cortisol imbalance;
5. Pregnancy and breastfeeding

Chapter 8: More about intermittent fasting

A very interesting topic to be discussed is what can be assumed in the hours of fasting, in fact, often we happen to read opinions and discordant opinions regarding this topic, but let's do a little clarity.

I try to deal with very complex topics in this chapter, writing them to make them suitable for everyone, trying to simplify technical notions and technical concepts; unfortunately when you make certain approximations you risk to flow into the "trivial" and say the crap, so I avoid going into too complicated speech providing only the bare minimum as the motivation of what I say.

To understand what foods can be consumed during fasting, we must understand the general concept of "being fasting".

In short, the "fasting" is a method of our organism to foresee the activation of some processes following the occurrence of some conditions, cause and effect.

What causes fasting is the energetic restriction in the short term and the glucidic restriction, hence two types of fasting are born, the intermittent one in which we talk about restricting the intervals of nutrition, and the carbohydrate fasting in which we limit the intake of carbohydrates for a few hours to bring to the surface the GLUT-4 receptors (they are carriers that carry glucose into the cell and are insulin-sensitive). During this period we perform a high enough refill to take advantage of the increased sensitivity to carbohydrates, gained in the fasting hours , these GLUT-4 are often the cause of the swelling that create carbohydrates; therefore the latter is also a very good strategy.

Both are fasting strategies, and can also be combined to improve their effects.

The effects of fasting are instead the activation of some metabolic pathways, such as the release of fatty acids for example, and the activation of catabolic processes in general, what we need to know is that these effects can be inhibited or enhanced on the basis of foods ingested, and that all the discourse goes a little way from the mere caloric value of what we eat!

We can distinguish 4 different categories for different types of drinks and effects they have on fasting:

okcal liquid foods that enhance the effects of fasting:

In this category we have foods like vinegar, coffee, green tea, black tea, multivitamin supplements (which I recommend to take with vegetables and not while fasting), water.

The stimulants, such as caffeine, which mediates the production of norepinephrine which mobilizes the glucose stocks and increasing the ADP / ATP ratio in turn activates AMPK / PPAR which is enough to let us know that they are all events that enhance the mobilization of acids fats and catabolic processes involved in fasting.

As for water, which is often not considered too much, drinking a good amount of water at once provokes an increase in pressure mediated by norepinephrine, which reconnected with what has been said about stimulants makes us realize that it has a very important.

Calorie liquid foods that enhance the effects of fasting:

Among the foods that we can consider with non-zero calories, we certainly find the famous BCAA (even if they are in powder, they are dissolved in water and therefore we consider them liquids), branched chain amino acids, even if they supply calories to our body, for a direct effect on limiting muscle catabolism (they are gluconeogenetic, they are used instead of amino acids derived from the "destruction" of muscle to produce glucose) provide benefits for fasting.

Another "surprise" food in this category is coconut oil. In fact, despite being a fat source and therefore very caloric, it does not stop glucose fasting, it activates the metabolic pathways that promote lipid oxidation, but being composed mostly of acids medium chain fat (MCT) will be very quickly (and most likely) addressed in mitochondria instead of being accumulated as fat.

Other similar foods are ghee or clarified butter, mostly

composed of MCT fats.

0kcal liquid foods that block the effects of fasting (or have no effect on the same):

There is not much to say about this category, because it should not even exist since there are practically no acaloric foods that block the fast, but only foods that have no effect on it, while not interrupting it. One example we could think of are sweeteners, but from several recent research releases, it has been noted that they have an (indirect) influence on the release of insulin, mediated by the perception of "sweet taste".

Obviously a few drops in coffee or tea will not block fasting, but it will not even have positive effects, they are "neutral".

An example of drinks are "zero" soda, which if you follow Martin Berkhan, you know you can take in quantity

Calorie liquid foods that block the effects of fasting:

Basically the most intuitive category; sugary drinks and liquid foods that bring more than 50kcal per 100g, if you like a drop of milk in the coffee, it will not be the one to block it (as long as it is a drop and not coffee milk)

For solid foods we have a greater limitation, practically there are foods that block fasting (caloric) and foods that enhance the effects (acaloric or limited calories <50kcal per 100g).

Foods that block fasting (calories):

All known and intuitive foods, cereals, sweets, dairy products, oils ... etc etc, in short, all the categories of foods that are excluded from fasting (using a little 'common sense can be easily understood).

Foods that enhance its effects (acaloric or limited calories <50kcal per 100g):

This is an interesting category, because we find very interesting foods, such as meat, for those who practice a PSMF (Protein Spared Modified Fast) is practically a fast in which they only take protein to limit muscle catabolism and spices; Among these we have cinnamon, black pepper, chilli pepper, turmeric. They are all spices that act on the factors of catabolism (the chili for example slightly increases the metabolism, making that the calories ingested are less than those necessary to digest it, fasting is a BOMB to enhance its effects).

Now that you know how to "create" the state of fasting, you can very well try experimenting combinations of various foods that will make it much more effective (and pleasant, like fasting coffee for example).

An example is that of the famous "Bulletproof coffee", MCT fats such as coconut oil or ghee (clarified butter) dissolved in hot coffee (or blended together), it may seem like rubbish but I assure you that it is a unique goodness, the foam that forms is a pleasure.

But even combinations like mint and cinnamon coffee, or mint tea and vanilla, are all tastes that we, as Westerners, are not used to and may seem strong or disgusting; but in the far east it has been used for centuries. If you are looking for some 0kcal recipe with coffee or tea, you will be amazed how simple it is to enjoy these drinks in countless different ways (and especially good), I recommend you try Turkish coffee , and I assure you that it will become a ritual to remain fasting just to savor its full taste!

As for intermittent fasting supplementation, practically all the supplements at 0kcal or that involve less than 50kcal per 100g are admitted (it is a value assigned by the office, it is not a magic rule, it is used to establish a range).

Multivitamins are good as well, but I recommend taking them with food as soon as the fast is broken because their absorption is greater when combined with high biological availability vitamins (such as those found in vegetables).

Another thing is to drink isotonic drinks. There is no problem as long as the total calories of the hiring drink are below the fateful 50kcal, so be sure to check the value of kcal that you take per serving before consuming the drink.

The same goes for pre workout blends and pre workout supplements in general (beta alanine, ALA, caffeine, creatine, taurine: everything is fine).

Chapter 9: How to deal with hunger attacks

With the term nervous hunger we mean the phenomenon for which a negative feeling in our mind unleashes a desire of unhealthy food that can not be managed.

The food chosen in this situation is the so-called "comfort food", or the foods very rich in sugar and fat, and the reason is a chemical one: the sudden rise of the level of sugar in the blood generates an immediate feeling of well-being and satisfaction. However, the sensation is only momentary and risks giving rise to that spiral of dependence on sugars that is the source of almost all hunger attacks of this type.

The reasons for the nervous hunger attacks are therefore to be found on a psychological level. Why do you eat when you're not really hungry? Because of boredom, sadness, anger, anxiety and other emotions. In short, we try to allay the negative feelings due to a work / family / sentimental issue with a food that ensures a momentary satisfaction.

How to control this attacks?

How to fight nervous hunger then? Here are some tips to put in place at the time of the nervous hunger attack and remedies to prevent it.

- The true cure of nervous hunger starts at the supermarket. It is important to make a clean house in the house of all those foods that our head requires in the moment of hunger attacks. It is not necessary, initially, to get rid of all "guilty" foods, but gradually start to buy less junk products (for example packaged ice creams, snacks, snacks, chips etc).

- Fill the fridge with healthy, easy-to-eat foods: fruits, raw vegetables, yogurt, etc.

- At the time of nervous hunger attacks try drinking lots of water or making herbal teas, perhaps choosing pleasing flavors like red fruits. Taking liquids will help you find a light feeling of fullness and satiety that can help you overcome the most acute moment of the hunger attack.

- In the same way you can go out for a walk, call a friend or a relative, arrange flowers and plants on the balcony, go to the gym or do another activity. In

71

short, you need to try something that you like, take your time or relax.

- Do not skip meals and always include vegetables, fruit and carbohydrates for lunch and dinner, preferably with a low glycemic index (for example whole wheat bread and pasta). Prolonged fasts and carbohydrate-free meals lower the level of sugar in the blood and this causes the brain to trigger mechanisms that induce the search for food and hence nervous hunger.

- Among the remedies for nervous hunger one of the most important one is to always have a snack in the morning and a snack in the afternoon. A good fruit, a yogurt, an orange juice, a tea with some dry biscuits or rusks, a fruit extract, a package of wholemeal crackers with low salt content, are all foods that help to get you hungry with meals.

- If the attacks are after dinner include an evening snack, in which you can eat the same foods listed for the morning snack. The important thing is that at least 2 hours have passed from dinner.

Here are other insightful tips that will allow you to avoid binge eating during the day.

- **Become smart like Sherlock Holmes!**

First of all, you must try to understand the situations that trigger hunger attacks. Maybe when you are under the pressure of exams and therefore very stressed? Or do you give up with a bar of chocolate every time the boss makes you nervous? Maybe when you're bored? Or is junk food just a way to console you when you're a bit off? Specifically rethink all the situations in which you succumbed to hunger attacks and look for a strategy to fight them. It's up to you to decide whether to rely on yoga to contain stress or change your job. What is certain is that you have to act and work on it, food can not be an outlet. Stress is closely linked to an unwanted increase in weight and certainly no one wants to get fat.

- **Break the routine and always choose the healthiest option**

It is not at all about eating only raw vegetables. On the contrary, it is necessary to consider every healthy choice that is made as part of a broader process of constant change, which allows us to avoid unhealthy foods from which we are often tempted, and to replace them with healthier options.

This is extremely important for two reasons: the first is that as soon as you adapt to a healthy diet, the change that occurs in your body is truly amazing. During the initial phase are changes that can not be seen because they mainly affect the complex metabolic processes of the body: for example, the hormones are secreted differently, the cells can become more sensitive to hormones and even taste buds become more sensitive to certain flavors. It is not uncommon for something that seems sweetened to the right point to become overly sweet just a few weeks after a healthier diet.

The second reason is that even that continuous desire for sweet snacks diminishes with time. If you're used to giving yourself sweet snacks a little too often in just one day, working on it a bit, you'll need it less and less: maybe just one day, yes and one, then once a week, until spending time you do not realize that, practically, it's something you do not do anymore. We are extremely routine based beings but habits can change. It only takes time.

- **Try some tricks**

If the snacks in which you want to sink your teeth every time you have a hunger attack are always on the desk, in the fridge at eye level or in view of the menu hanging from the fridge, it becomes very difficult to resist and win temptations. As they say: when eye does not see, heart does not hurt. If there is nothing that can tempt you near you, do not take that automatism for which you see something that engulfs you and you eat it without even thinking about it. It is obvious that the best thing would be to have none of the foods that usually make you gorge at your fingertips. Not surprisingly, if you have to go to the supermarket to satisfy a hunger attack, there is a very high probability that you can resist.

- **Dab hunger attacks with artificial sweeteners**

In short: artificial sweeteners (such as aspartame, saccharin and company) do not do well. Because? If you continue to consume extremely sweet foods, you will never be able to adapt to a normal degree of sweetness. Furthermore, it has been scientifically proven that eating sweet food without calories in it triggers an even stronger desire for sweetness, which means that after a snack containing artificial sweeteners is consumed, there is a risk that you may want to eat an extra bar of chocolate. This is how temptation wins once again. Finally, many studies have shown that people who regularly consume artificial sweeteners, such as cola light, have a higher chance of gaining weight and developing type 2 diabetes.

So what can you eat when a hunger attack comes?

Here the question becomes really interesting. What can you eat when a hunger attack comes? You have to keep some things in mind when choosing a snack.

Choose foods rich in nutrients and high in fiber. They guarantee a good sense of satiety and often have a better calorie / quantity ratio compared to industrial snacks. You can choose for example fruits with a low content of natural sugars such as berries, grapefruit or avocado. Even a handful of nuts, a piece of dark chocolate or dried dates are a good option. Remember though that it is not good to even abuse healthy snacks, because in some cases they have a lot of calories (take for example nuts or avocados).

However, if you really want to lose weight, try to opt as much as possible for foods with very few calories, so you do not have limits in terms of quantity, thanks to the richness of fiber and low calories. You can choose from: peppers, kohlrabi, tomatoes, cucumbers, mushrooms, salad, radishes, beets and broccoli. The word chocolate certainly sounds more inviting, but over time you will learn to love these snacks too. And remember, "no pain - no gain".

Let's recap our golden rules.

- Become smart as Sherlock Holmes: investigate the causes that trigger your hunger attacks and then work on it!
- Break the routine: try to eat less frequently between main meals.
- Try a few tricks: avoid having snacks at your fingertips and try not to buy unhealthy ones.
- Do not eat foods that contain artificial sweeteners.
- Drink a glass of fresh water before eating. This fact can give you a first sense of satiety.
- When choosing a snack, always opt for the healthiest: choose fruit with low sugar content or raw vegetables.
- Eat slowly and consciously. Focus on what you eat and avoid doing other things like working or watching TV.

- Take your time. The sense of satiety always makes us feel a bit. Be patient.

- Exercise! Physical activity helps to eliminate stress, distract and strengthen the body. It's always a great idea, is not it?

- Willpower! It is not easy, but nobody said it would be. So be strong and trust yourself!

Conclusion

Thank for making it through to the end of this book, let's hope it was informative and able to provide you with all of the tools you need to achieve your goals whatever it is that they may be. Just because you've finished this book doesn't mean there is nothing left to learn on the topic, expanding your horizons is the only way to find the mastery you seek.

The next step is to stop reading and to get starting doing whatever it is that you need to do in order to ensure that you are able to get amazing results with intermittent fasting. If you find that you still need help getting started you will likely have better results by creating a schedule that you hope to follow including strict deadlines for various parts of the tasks as well as the overall completion of your preparations.

Studies show that complex tasks that are broken down into individual pieces, including individual deadlines, have a much greater chance of being completed when compared to something that has a general need of being completed but no real time table for doing so. Even if it seems silly, go ahead and set your own deadlines for completion, complete with indicators of success and failure. After you have successfully completed all of your required preparations you will be glad you did. For example, you can think about practicing one new intermittent fasting food habit every day, before becoming a general master of the diet. It is your choice and it is the beauty of dieting and cooking.

Once you have tried the same recipe many times, it is the right moment to invite your friends and ask them to try the intermittent fasting diet: they are going to love it and, best of all, see incredible results with it.